BEGINNER GUIDE TO TAI CHI FOR STRESS REDUCTION

Unlock Inner Peace With Mindfulness Practice, Anxiety Reduction, Relaxation Techniques, Meditation Exercises And Holistic Wellness Strategies

MALCOLM KASHTON

DISCLAIMER

This book contains information that is solely meant to be used for educational and informative reasons. This includes training regimens, game strategy, and fitness recommendations. Despite having taken every precaution to guarantee the correctness and completeness of the material provided, the author disclaims all express and implied warranties and representations regarding the content's suitability, timeliness, reliability, or accuracy for any purpose.

This book's content is not meant to be a replacement for expert medical advice, diagnosis, or care. When in doubt about a medical problem, never hesitate to consult your doctor or another trained healthcare professional. Never ignore medical advice from professionals or put off getting it because of something you've read in this book.

The material provided here and how you utilize it are not the responsibility of the author or publisher. You bear full responsibility for any reliance you make on the information contained in this book. The publisher and author disclaim all liability for any loss or damage resulting from using this book, including but not limited to indirect or consequential loss or damage, or any loss or damage from losing data or profits.

All references in this book to particular goods, services, or organizations are made for informative purposes only and do not imply endorsement or recommendation on the part of the publisher or author.

You acknowledge that there is no responsibility for any harm or injury that may arise from utilizing the material in this book, and that you will hold the author and publisher harmless by reading and using it. You alone are in charge of your own health and wellbeing, so you should apply any advice or suggestions from this book with caution and good judgment.

Table Of Contents

ABOUT THE BOOK

"Tai Chi for Stress Reduction," provides a thorough explanation of how to practice Tai Chi to understand and manage stress. The book's goal is stated at the outset by the author, who also highlights the real-world advantages of Tai Chi for stress relief. The preface offers instructions to readers on how to get the most out of the book.

The basic idea of stress is explored, along with its definition and consequences on the body and mind. After that, the story moves smoothly to explain how important Tai Chi is for stress relief.

Readers are given a comprehensive overview of Tai Chi, including its history, origins, and basic concepts, as well as an outline of the various forms that make up this age-old Chinese martial art. As a helpful manual for novices, the book explains basic movements, helps them select the appropriate Tai Chi style, and emphasizes the significance of correct breathing techniques.

The relationship between Tai Chi and mindfulness is examined, with a focus on how the body and mind work together in the practice. Readers are provided with a comprehensive approach to stress reduction through the meticulously defined techniques for relaxation, tension release, and meditation found in Tai Chi.

Building a regular Tai Chi practice, dealing with typical problems, and offering direction on advancing in the Tai Chi journey are all covered. The book is customizing Tai Chi exercises for various types of stress, such as relationship stress, work-related stress, and daily pressures.

The book takes readers into more advanced territory by introducing advanced Tai Chi techniques. It also encourages readers to explore more complex motions and apply Tai Chi to their daily lives to enhance their practice. By emphasizing the connections between Tai Chi, yoga, and meditation, it broadens the scope and provides a comprehensive stress-reduction strategy that incorporates complementary activities.

"Tai Chi for Stress Reduction" is an invaluable tool for anyone looking for a realistic and comprehensive method of using the age-old practice of Tai Chi to manage stress. From comprehending stress to using sophisticated strategies, the book offers a well-organized approach that enables readers to develop a harmonious balance between their bodily and mental well-being.

CHAPTER ONE

OVERVIEW OF TAI CHI FOR STRESS REDUCTION

TAI CHI'S STRESS-REDUCTION BENEFITS

Stress has become an unavoidable aspect of our everyday lives in this fast-paced and demanding society, negatively affecting our mental and physical health. Stress can take many different forms and intensities, but it is commonly understood to be the body's reaction to any change that necessitates adjustment or response. Many people experience high levels of stress as a result of the constant demands of modern life, including social expectations, personal struggles, and professional obligations.

Understanding the tremendous effects that long-term stress may have on the body and mind is crucial.

RECOGNIZING STRESS

Simply put, stress is the body's response to something it perceives as a threat or demand. A series of physiological reactions, including the production of stress hormones like cortisol and adrenaline, are set off by this reaction. While temporary stress can be a healthy and adaptive response, long-term stress exposure without enough recuperation might have negative health repercussions. The consequences of stress transcend beyond mental and emotional health to encompass multiple physiological systems, with the potential to exacerbate cardiovascular problems, impaired immune response, and heightened vulnerability to diverse ailments.

THE MEANING OF STRESS

Tai Chi is a complex kind of exercise that has become known as a comprehensive method of reducing stress. Tai Chi is a form of martial arts that has its roots in ancient China. It is distinguished by its methodical, slow movements, controlled breathing, and contemplative mental state. Together, these components support the body's natural energy flow, which creates equilibrium and tranquility. As a mindfulness exercise, tai chi helps people to concentrate their attention away from worries and become present in the moment.

There are several advantages to practicing Tai Chi for lowering stress. Tai Chi's soft, regular movements ease muscle tension and encourage relaxation, which lessens the physical effects of stress. By promoting deep, diaphragmatic breathing, the physiological impacts of the stress response are lessened and respiratory function is improved. In addition, Tai Chi's meditative component fosters mental clarity and mindfulness while providing practitioners with a break from the never-ending demands of everyday life.

STRESS'S IMPACT ON THE BODY AND MIND

Comprehending the complex relationship between stress and the body is essential to realizing the potential benefits of stress-reduction techniques like Tai Chi. A wide range of health problems, including immune system impairment, sleeplessness, and hypertension, have been connected to chronic stress. People can actively mitigate these negative effects and develop a more resilient reaction to stressors by practicing Tai Chi regularly.

TAI CHI'S FUNCTION IN STRESS REDUCTION

Tai Chi shows itself as a potent instrument that goes beyond simple physical exercise in the field of stress management. Because of its holistic approach, which tackles stress from both a physical and psychological perspective, it's a useful and approachable technique for anyone looking for a complete stress-reduction plan. By incorporating Tai Chi into daily routines, we may create a haven of calm amid the chaos of modern life, supporting not only physical health but also mental toughness in the face of adversity.

CHAPTER TWO

AN OVERVIEW OF TAI CHI

TAI CHI'S ORIGINS & HISTORY

Tai Chi is an ancient Chinese martial art with roots in Taoism and other Chinese philosophies. It is also known as Tai Chi Chuan or Taijiquan. It is thought to have been built by Chen Wangting in Chen Village, Henan Province, in the seventeenth century. According to legend, Chen was motivated to combine the spiritual and physical elements of martial arts by the movements of animals and the concepts of Yin and Yang. Tai Chi changed over time from being a martial art to a comprehensive discipline that included self-defense, meditation, and wellness.

Different types and interpretations of Tai Chi arose as the art form spread throughout China, each adding to its rich tapestry. Yang Luchan altered the Chen style in the 19th century to produce what is today called Yang-style Tai Chi.

Other styles followed, each with distinct shapes and traits, including the Wu, Hao, and Sun styles. The development of tai chi from a remote village tradition to a worldwide phenomenon is evidence of its versatility and allure.

FUNDAMENTALS OF TAI CHI

Fundamental concepts form the foundation of Tai Chi and influence both its philosophy and practice. The idea of Yin and Yang, which stands for the dualities of nature and life, is one of the fundamental ideas. Tai Chi places a strong emphasis on the harmonic balancing of opposing forces—whether they be forceful and yielding, soft and hard, or slow and quick. By fostering a condition of dynamic balance, practitioners want to facilitate the smooth movement of energy, or "Qi," throughout the body.

A further fundamental idea is the development of internal strength, or "Neijin." Tai Chi stresses internal power produced by good body alignment, relaxation, and controlled breathing, in contrast to exterior martial arts that emphasize muscular strength. Tai Chi's core idea is "song," which refers to unwinding or releasing unneeded stress. Maintaining a state of relaxation helps practitioners become more attuned to the flow of energy and cultivates a flexible, adaptable body.

The practices of mindfulness and meditation are essential to Tai Chi. The artwork promotes mental clarity and presence by keeping the mind quiet and concentrated. Through the execution of movements with heightened awareness, practitioners can establish connections with both their inner selves and the surrounding environment. Tai Chi transforms into a form of moving meditation that encourages balance and calmness in the body and mind.

DIFFERENT TAI CHI STYLES

Different Tai Chi styles have developed throughout the years, each with its forms, distinctive qualities, and emphasis on specific principles. Among the most popular styles are:

• Chen Style: This original form, which originated in Chen Village, is distinguished by a fusion of fluid, leisurely motion, and sudden, intense energy bursts. It combines harsh and soft aspects, which makes it a lively and difficult style of Tai Chi.

• Yang Style: The most popular and well-known style was developed by Yang Luchan. It is suitable for people of all ages and fitness levels because it stresses relaxation and has calm, elegant motions.

Wu Jianquan is credited with creating the Wu Style, which is distinguished by its elegant and compact movements. It emphasizes the internal aspects of Tai Chi, including the cultivation of Qi and the exact alignment of the body.

• Hao Style: Known for its deliberate, tiny motions, the Hao style is among the rarest and oldest forms of Tai

Chi. It emphasizes specific skills, attention, and inner power.

- Sun Style: Developed by Sun Lutang, this form incorporates ideas from different martial arts along with traditional Tai Chi techniques. It highlights a more natural and erect posture and integrates nimble footwork.

Every style provides a unique method of practicing tai chi, meeting the requirements, interests, and skill levels of many people. All Tai Chi styles aim to promote mental and physical well-being as well as a greater comprehension of the concepts of harmony and balance, even though their forms and techniques may differ.

CHAPTER THREE

TAI CHI AS A STRESS-REDUCTION TECHNIQUE

TAI CHI RELAXATION TECHNIQUES

The ancient Chinese martial art of tai chi is well known for its significant effects on relaxation and general well-being. Its ideology revolves around the development of a serene state of mind. A fundamental aspect of Tai Chi relaxation is matching deep, diaphragmatic breathing with soft, flowing motions. This synchronization facilitates relaxation on both the physical and mental levels by fostering a sense of connection between the mind and body.

Tai Chi practitioners are encouraged to focus on the present moment through deliberate and slow movements, which cultivates mindfulness. People can progressively release tension and stress by focusing on the minute changes in body weight and the smoothness of each movement.

The focus on mindfulness in Tai Chi is a potent relaxation technique that helps practitioners let go of outside worries and lose themselves in the rhythmic flow of the form.

RELEASING STRESS USING TAI CHI FORMS

Tai Chi movements emphasize a smooth transition from one position to the next and are distinguished by their elegant, continuous flow. This methodical approach to movement is a useful way to relieve stress that has built up in the muscles and joints. Tai Chi promotes a sensation of suppleness and flexibility by gradually releasing physical stiffness through regulated motions and gentle stretches.

In Tai Chi, the idea of "sung" is essential for relieving tension. Sung, which is frequently translated as "relaxation," is a special kind of rest that combines mental and physical calm. It is advised of practitioners to keep their minds clear and attentive while simultaneously relaxing their muscles and joints.

This combination releases tension and encourages a relaxed, centered state by facilitating the free passage of energy (Qi) throughout the body.

INCLUDING MEDITATION IN TAI CHI PRACTICE

In the context of Tai Chi, relaxation is greatly enhanced by meditation. Clear, peaceful mental states and focused breath awareness are frequently experienced in tandem with slow, purposeful movements. This contemplative feature invites practitioners to focus inside, developing a close relationship with their bodies and breath.

During the practice of Tai Chi meditation, one must develop an attitude of mindfulness and attentiveness. People can let go of their thoughts and outside distractions by focusing on the here and now, which makes it possible for a deep sense of relaxation to be established. Tai Chi is a holistic approach to general well-being since it incorporates meditation into the practice, which not only improves physical relaxation but also fosters mental clarity and emotional equilibrium.

The relaxation techniques found in Tai Chi include the deliberate release of physical tension through flowing postures, the synchronization of movements with deep breathing, and the integration of meditation for an increased level of mindfulness. By using these tenets, Tai Chi offers a thorough method of relaxation that encourages balance and harmony in the body and mind.

CHAPTER FOUR

HOW TO BEGIN LEARNING TAI CHI

SELECTING YOUR IDEAL TAI CHI STYLE

Choosing a Tai Chi style that suits your goals, preferences, and physical condition is one of the most important decisions you will make when you first start. There are many different types of tai chi, each with its foundational ideas and techniques. The most popular styles, which are distinguished by particular forms and methods, are Yang, Chen, Wu, Sun, and Hao. Beginners prefer the Yang style because of its flowing, soft motions, while those looking for a more dynamic practice will find the Chen style, which combines slow and explosive movements, intriguing. By investigating the ideas and traits of each style, you can make an informed decision about which one best suits your goals and sense of self.

FUNDAMENTAL POSTURES AND MOVEMENTS IN TAI CHI

You must comprehend the basic postures and motions of Tai Chi before diving in. The slow, methodical motions of tai chi are well known for encouraging balance, coordination, and a harmonious flow of energy. Stability and relaxation are based on fundamental postures, like "Wuji" or the preparation pose. The typical motions "Grasp the Sparrow's Tail" and "Golden Rooster Stands on One Leg" highlight precise alignment, weight shifting, and smooth transitions. In addition to improving the physical benefits of Tai Chi, mastering these fundamentals paves the way for more complex forms and sequences that appear as you advance in your practice.

THE VALUE OF APPROPRIATE BREATHING

It is impossible to emphasize how important adequate breathing is to Tai Chi. a fundamental component of this traditional Chinese martial art and holistic practice is the incorporation of breathing into movement. Breathing in a deep, slow, and attentive manner has several benefits: it eases stress, strengthens the bond between the body and mind, and allows Qi, the life energy, to flow freely. The focus is on diaphragmatic breathing, which increases lung capacity and oxygenates the body by having the abdomen expand and contract with each breath. Breath-movement synchronization soothes the nervous system and improves practice effectiveness, allowing for a more in-depth investigation of the mind-body relationship. Developing an awareness of your breath and using it in your Tai Chi practice will enhance its overall health benefits and make it a more meaningful and satisfying practice.

CHAPTER FIVE

DEVELOPING YOUR TAI CHI PRACTICE

ESTABLISHING A REGULAR PRACTICE SCHEDULE

Developing a regular practice schedule for Tai Chi is essential to fully benefiting from this age-old Chinese martial art. Start by establishing attainable goals that complement your specific ambitions and degree of fitness.

Customizing your routine to meet your unique needs promotes a more sustainable practice, whether your goals are to improve your physical well-being, lower your stress level, or develop mindfulness.

Regularity is equally as important as session length in achieving consistency. Make Tai Chi a regular part of your routine by scheduling it into your daily or weekly routine. This can entail setting up a particular period, like the mornings or the nights, to focus on your practice. By incorporating Tai Chi into your everyday routine, you provide the groundwork for sustained dedication and advancement.

OVERCOMING TYPICAL OBSTACLES

Starting a Tai Chi journey can present some difficulties, but knowing what to expect can help you get through them successfully. When facing the early learning curve, patience is essential because it takes time and perseverance to become proficient in Tai Chi motions. Overcoming frustration and despair might be aided by acknowledging that progress is sluggish.

Striking the correct balance between rest and focus is another frequent problem. Achieving the special balance of focus and suppleness required for Tai Chi can be difficult.

Achieving this equilibrium necessitates self-awareness and mindfulness, which enable practitioners to continuously modify and improve their strategy.

Another problem is incorporating Tai Chi into a hectic lifestyle. To get around this, think about quick, concentrated sessions that you can fit right into your everyday schedule. You may make the exercise more accessible and ensure that your progress is not impeded by a hectic schedule by breaking it down into smaller segments.

MOVING FORWARD WITH YOUR TAI CHI PRACTICE

Gaining proficiency in Tai Chi is more than just physical skill; it's a dynamic and individual journey. Develop a mindset that values lifelong learning and sees every practice session as a chance to improve. Return to the basics often to hone your comprehension of the postures, moves, and tenets of Tai Chi.

Learn more by investigating the origins and philosophy of Tai Chi. Gaining an understanding of the cultural background and guiding ideas can improve your experience in general and strengthen your bond with the practice. Participate in seminars and workshops or ask knowledgeable teachers for advice to improve your skills and acquire insightful knowledge.

To push you farther as you grow, think about adding variants and advanced forms. Adapt your practice to your changing objectives, whether they are to become healthier, become more proficient in your form, or explore the deeper spiritual side of Tai Chi. Recognize and celebrate the minor wins along the way as your form, balance, and general well-being improve subtly. This all-encompassing strategy makes sure that your experience with Tai Chi is sustainable and satisfying in the long run.

CHAPTER SIX

MINDFULNESS AND TAI CHI

LINKING THE MIND AND BODY

The ancient Chinese martial arts and mindfulness practice of tai chi places a strong focus on mind-body integration. Tai Chi is based on the fundamental idea that physical and mental health are interdependent and that maintaining their balance is crucial to general well-being. Tai Chi's leisurely, flowing movements are a means by which practitioners can develop a more acute awareness of their mental and physical conditions. Breath and movement synchronization allows practitioners to explore the body's subtle sensations mindfully and strengthens the bond between their mental and physical selves.

OBSERVANT FORM IN TAI CHI:

The idea of attentive movement lies at the core of Tai Chi practice. Tai Chi teaches practitioners to move with a purposeful and mindful awareness of each motion, in contrast to many other forms of physical exercise. People can cultivate mindfulness by focusing on the present moment through the deliberate and slow motions of Tai Chi. By paying careful attention to posture, how weight is distributed, and how smoothly transitions occur, practitioners can reach a profound state of concentration that strengthens the mind's ability to be present in the moment. As a result, Tai Chi turns into a form of moving meditation that enhances calmness and mindfulness.

GAINING MINDFULNESS BY PRACTICING TAI CHI

Tai Chi is an effective method for fostering mindfulness because it provides a disciplined environment in which people can practice raising their level of awareness. To cultivate a nonjudgmental awareness of thoughts and emotions, the practice entails a purposeful transfer of focus from exterior distractions to internal sensations. Practitioners can release tension, worry, and obsessions as they become attentive to the present moment through the flowing, rhythmic motions. Tai Chi's meditation component helps people cultivate a mindful attitude toward obstacles, both on and off the practice mat, which fosters a sense of composed resilience in the face of life's difficulties.

Being conscious is not an isolated activity in Tai Chi; rather, it is an essential component of the form. By practicing deliberate, slow movements regularly, practitioners progressively improve their capacity to sustain a heightened awareness in daily life. The concepts of Tai Chi transcend the material world; they impact how people confront difficulties, relate to others, and negotiate the intricacies of their inner selves. Thus, including mindfulness in Tai Chi practice creates a life-changing experience that promotes a harmonious body-mind connection that goes well beyond the practice area.

CHAPTER SEVEN
ADVANCED FORMS OF TAI CHI
ENHANCING YOUR FORM OF TAI CHI

To improve your Tai Chi practice, you must go beyond the basic forms and comprehend the fundamental ideas that underpin this age-old martial art. Cultivating a strong feeling of awareness is one important component.

As you advance, concentrate on the internal elements of Tai Chi, such as your breathing, the flow of energy, and the relationship between your body and mind. A more comprehensive approach to the exercise is encouraged by mindful awareness, which amplifies the efficiency of every movement.

Improving your body mechanics is another essential component of developing your Tai Chi practice. Be very aware of your alignment, weight distribution, and posture.

By refining these principles, you can make sure that the energy produced by every action is distributed evenly, which promotes control and balance. Accepting the nuances of body alignment and weight shifts helps you become more proficient and adds to the overall flow of your Tai Chi form.

EXAMINING COMPLEX MOTIONS

Beyond the fundamental forms, advanced Tai Chi moves to provide complex patterns and combinations that test your physical and mental limits. The "Push Hands" technique is one such advanced movement that combines partner exercises to improve balance, responsiveness, and sensitivity. By practicing Push Hands, practitioners can delve deeper into the subtleties of energy interaction and gain a better grasp of the martial applications of Tai Chi.

One more feature of advanced Tai Chi is the use of silk-reeling movements. The smooth circulation of energy throughout the body is facilitated by these continual, spiraling motions. Learning silk-reeling methods improves a practitioner's general coordination and fluidity, which helps them perform more difficult Tai Chi sequences with grace and ease.

INCLUDING TAI CHI IN EVERYDAY ACTIVITIES

Tai Chi is a way of life, and its core goes beyond the four walls of a practice session. Embracing the concepts of awareness, balance, and relaxation in every moment is essential to incorporating tai chi into everyday activities. Start by using the concepts of Tai Chi for basic movements such as sitting, standing, and walking. Develop a sense of grounded awareness so that, even when engaging in daily tasks, the mind and body remain connected.

Moreover, practicing Tai Chi regularly calls for developing a thoughtful stress-reduction strategy. Apply the concepts of Tai Chi to deal with situations in a composed and collected manner.

Tai Chi can be practiced as a guiding principle to promote a harmonious and balanced existence, whether in job or personal connections. The benefits of Tai Chi can be extended beyond the practice area by regularly incorporating these ideas into your daily routine, leading to a more complete and transforming way of life.

CHAPTER EIGHT

TAI CHI FOR PARTICULAR STRESSES

TAI CHI FOR STRESS AT WORK

The ancient Chinese martial art of tai chi, which has developed into a comprehensive fitness regimen, has significant advantages in reducing stress associated with a range of issues, including relationships, the workplace, and daily obstacles. It is an effective technique for enhancing mental, emotional, and physical well-being because of its thoughtful, flowing motions.

Tai Chi offers a special and useful way to combat the stress of a hectic and demanding work environment when it comes to work-related stress. Tai Chi's methodical, slow movements combined with purposeful breathing exercises help people relax, straighten their posture, and become more aware of their bodies. Practitioners can improve concentration, better handle workplace stress, and encourage a more balanced approach to their professional responsibilities by developing a sense of calm and focus.

TAI CHI FOR STRESS IN RELATIONSHIPS

Stressful relationships can hurt a person's physical and emotional well-being, which can affect how they interact with other people. With its focus on balance and harmony, tai chi can be a helpful exercise for couples trying to work through difficulties.

Partners can develop a closer bond and enhance communication by moving in unison and focusing on each other. The meditative elements of Tai Chi also help people become more self-aware, which helps them control their emotional responses and develop a more understanding and caring interpersonal style.

TAI CHI FOR TYPICAL STRESS ISSUES

Tai Chi offers a flexible way to deal with life's ups and downs and every day worries. Because of its flexibility, practitioners may easily include it in their daily schedules, whether they use it as a quick break during a busy day or as a morning habit. The body and mind are engaged by the slow, rhythmic motions, which encourage relaxation and lessen the physiological effects of stress. Regular Tai Chi practice promotes a conscious way of living, building resilience and a positive outlook that can help one respond to life's obstacles in a more balanced way.

Tai Chi is essentially a holistic practice that attends to the interrelated domains of mental, emotional, and physical health. People can gain useful abilities to manage and lessen tensions connected to work, relationships, and the numerous obstacles that come up in daily life by implementing Tai Chi into their daily routines. The balancing concepts of Tai Chi provide a technique to build resilience, improve the general quality of life, and encourage a well-rounded strategy for negotiating the intricacies of today's society.

CHAPTER NINE

USING TAI CHI IN CONJUNCTION WITH OTHER STRESS-REDUCTION METHODS

COMBINING YOGA, MEDITATION, AND TAI CHI

By combining Tai Chi, yoga, and meditation, three age-old traditions that all aim to enhance mind-body harmony are brought together. The Chinese martial art of tai chi places a strong emphasis on deep breathing and fluid, leisurely motions.

These techniques work best when combined with yoga's gentle postures and deliberate breathing, which promotes a holistic approach to stress relief. Tai Chi's meditative component complements meditation well, adding to the overall relaxing effect on the mind. When combined, these techniques produce a synergistic effect that enhances emotional equilibrium, mental clarity, and physical health.

EXAMINING SUPPLEMENTARY METHODS

When it comes to reducing stress, experimenting with supplementary methods in addition to Tai Chi offers a wide variety of choices to address different facets of well-being. To maximize the stress-relieving effects of Tai Chi, mindfulness exercises like progressive muscular relaxation and deep breathing exercises can be smoothly included in the program. Furthermore, Qigong, which has roots in Tai Chi, is a practice that can enhance and complement it. By combining these techniques, people can customize their stress-reduction plan to meet their requirements and preferences, resulting in a comprehensive and flexible approach.

MAKING A COMPREHENSIVE PLAN FOR STRESS REDUCTION

To address the complex nature of stress, a comprehensive stress reduction plan should incorporate Tai Chi with a range of complementary treatments. Along with Tai Chi, adding yoga, deep breathing techniques, and mindfulness meditation to the practice offers a complete arsenal for stress management on the mental, emotional, and physical levels.

A holistic approach acknowledges that stress impacts various facets of an individual's being and, hence, demands a comprehensive approach. People can develop a robust mind-body connection and promote overall well-being in addition to stress reduction by integrating these several disciplines.

Beyond physical activities, the holistic stress reduction strategy takes into account lifestyle elements like getting enough sleep, eating a healthy diet, and maintaining social relationships. A proactive, all-encompassing approach to stress management is encouraged when Tai Chi is incorporated into a larger wellness framework. This comprehensive approach acknowledges the interdependence of diverse facets of health and enables people to adopt lifestyle decisions that enhance their general well-being.

Essentially, combining Tai Chi with other methods of stress reduction opens the door to a more all-encompassing and long-term strategy for handling the pressures of contemporary life.

CHAPTER TEN

PROSPECTIVE PATTERNS AND ADVANCEMENTS IN SPORTS WELL-BEING

PROGRESS IN THE FIELD OF FUNCTIONAL MEDICINE

Developments in functional medicine are fundamentally changing the way that athletes are well. While functional medicine adopts a holistic approach by addressing the underlying causes of health disorders, traditional medicine frequently concentrates on treating symptoms. This strategy seeks to maximize overall well-being while taking into account the interdependence of different body systems. Functional medicine is becoming more well-known in the area of athlete wellness due to its integrative and individualized approaches. Through the integration of targeted therapies, lifestyle adjustments, and nutrition, athletes can get both improved performance and long-term health advantages.

NEW TECHNOLOGIES

The way that athletes track and maintain their health is being completely transformed by emerging technologies. Smartwatches and fitness trackers are examples of wearable technology that is getting more and more advanced. These gadgets can provide real-time information on vital signs, sleep patterns, and physical activity. Athletes and their medical teams can use this information to make well-informed decisions on training plans, recuperation techniques, and injury prevention.

Athletes' cognitive abilities are also improved by using innovations like virtual reality (VR) and augmented reality (AR) for mental training and recovery. These technological advancements are helping to advance athlete wellness through a more thorough and customized approach.

DEVELOPING THE FUTURE OF HEALTHCARE FOR ATHLETES

A paradigm change in favor of proactive and preventive interventions is required to shape the future of athlete healthcare. The emphasis is on preserving good health and avoiding problems before they exist, as opposed to only treating illnesses and injuries after they occur. Regular health examinations, individualized diet regimens, and proactive injury prevention techniques are all part of this proactive strategy. Healthcare providers can design customized wellness plans for athletes by combining data from wearables and sophisticated tests. Additionally, the combined efforts of sports medicine specialists, dietitians, psychologists, and other professionals result in a multidisciplinary approach that takes into account every aspect of the well-being of athletes.

The combination of these factors points to an all-encompassing strategy for athlete wellness that goes beyond traditional approaches.

Emerging technologies that offer real-time insights into an athlete's physiology are integrated with functional medicine to enhance its individualized care philosophy. A proactive approach to athlete healthcare that makes use of wearable technology, sophisticated diagnostics, and teamwork to maximize performance, avoid injuries, and increase general well-being is the way of the future. Athletes may anticipate a more thorough and individualized approach to their health as these trends develop, guaranteeing a long-lasting and fruitful career in sports.